The Last Keto Diet Cakes Recipe Book

Enjoy your Keto Cakes while Losing Weight with the Power of Keto Diet

Jessica Simpson

Contents

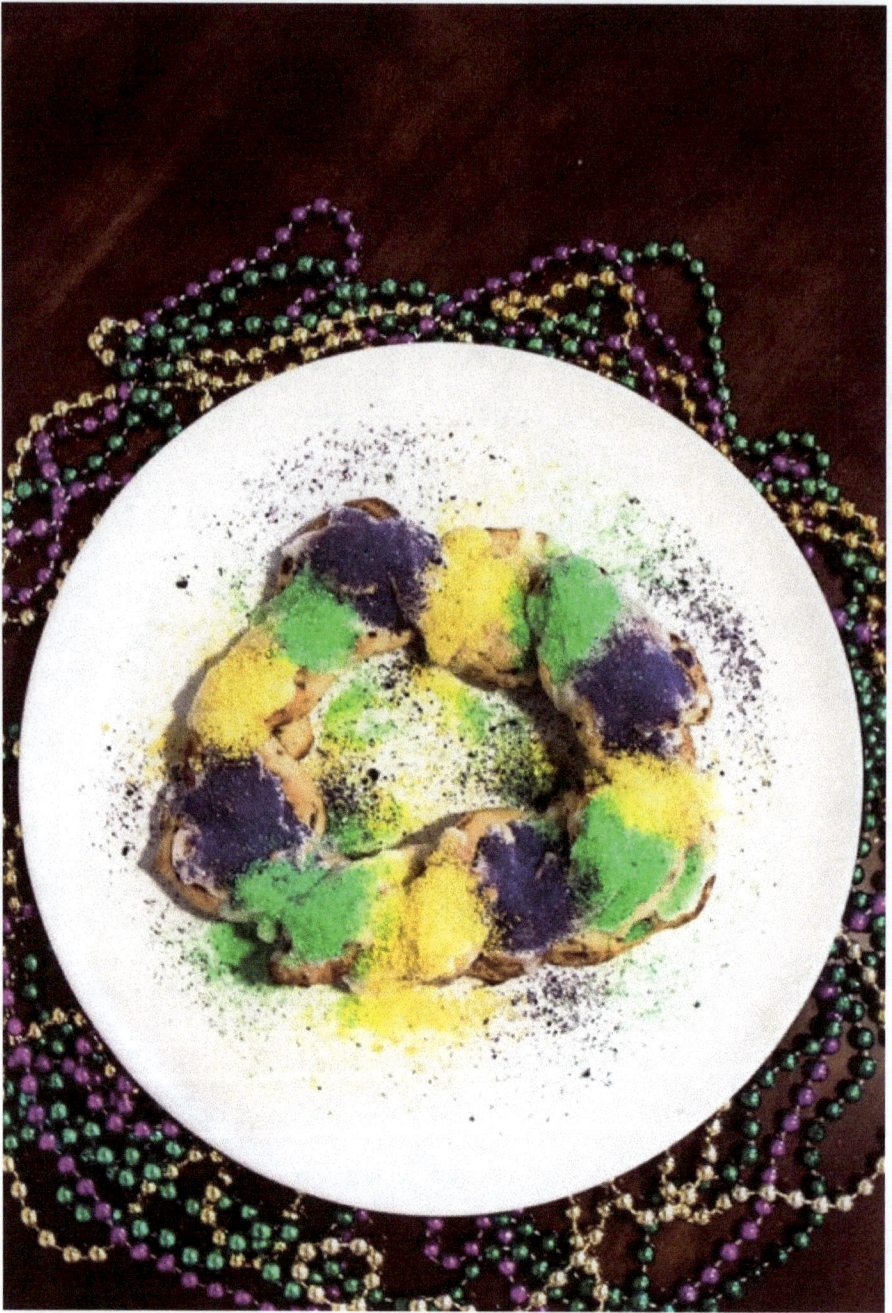

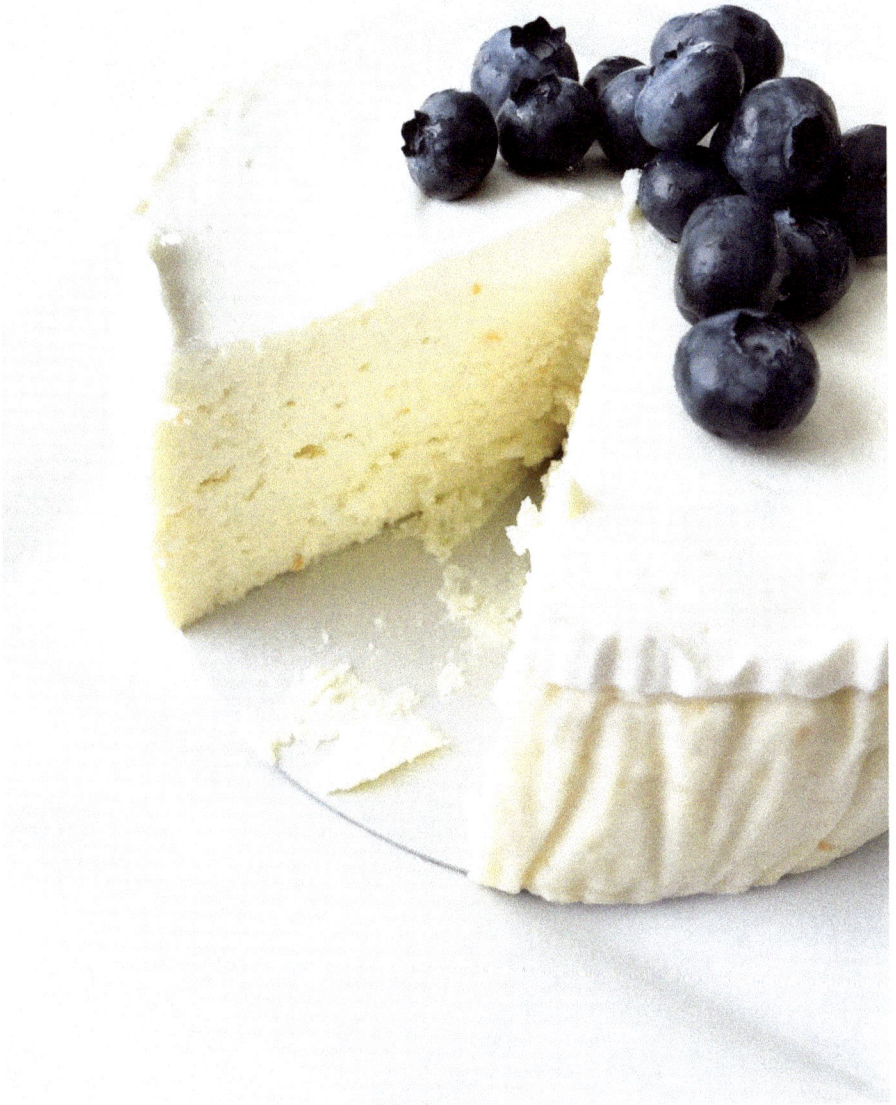

Cake With Whipped Cream Icing

Servings: 7

Cooking Time: 25 Minutes

Ingredients:

- ¾ Cup Coconut flour
- ¾ Cup of Swerve Sweetener
- ½ Cup of Cocoa powder
- 2 Teaspoons of Baking powder
- 6 Large Eggs
- 2/3 Cup of Heavy Whipping Cream
- ½ Cup of Melted almond Butter
- For the whipped Cream Icing:
- 1 Cup of Heavy Whipping Cream
- ¼ Cup of Swerve Sweetener
- 1 Teaspoon of Vanilla extract
- 1/3 Cup of Sifted Cocoa Powder

Directions:

1. Pre-heat your oven to a temperature of about 350 F.
2. Grease an 8x8 cake tray with cooking spray.
3. Add the coconut flour, the Swerve sweetener; the cocoa powder, the baking powder, the eggs, the melted butter; and combine very well with an electric or a hand mixer.

4. Pour your batter into the cake tray and bake for about 25 minutes.

5. Remove the cake tray from the oven and let cool for about minutes.

6. For the Icing

7. Whip the cream until it becomes fluffy; then add in the Swerve, the vanilla and the cocoa powder.

8. Add the Swerve, the vanilla and the cocoa powder; then continue mixing until your ingredients are very well combined.

9. Frost your baked cake with the icing; then slice it; serve and enjoy your delicious cake!

Nutrition Info: Calories: 357;Fat: 33g;Carbohydrates: 11g;Fiber: 2g;Protein: 8g

Spiced Stewed Rhubarb

Servings: 4

Cooking Time:30 Minutes

Ingredients:

- 3 cups chopped fresh rhubarb
- 1 tsp Stevia/your preferred keto sweetener
- 1 tsp vanilla extract
- Juice of ½ lemon
- 3 Tbsp butter
- 1 cup water

Directions:

1. Place all ingredients into a large saucepan and place over a medium heat
2. Bring the mixture to boiling point then reduce to a simmer
3. Allow the mixture to simmer away until the rhubarb is nice and soft and the liquids have reduced
4. Store in an airtight jar in the fridge until required!

Nutrition Info: Calories: 100 ;Fat: 9 grams ;Protein: 1 gram ;Total carbs: 3 grams ;Net carbs: 3 grams

Fudgy R18 Sauce

Servings: 5

Cooking Time: 20 Minutes

Ingredients:

- 4 oz 72% cocoa dark chocolate
- 1 cup heavy cream
- 2 Tbsp cocoa powder
- ½ tsp Stevia/your preferred keto sweetener
- 3 Tbsp dark rum
- Pinch of sea salt

Directions:

1. Place the chocolate and cream into a heatproof bowl over a saucepan of water and stir as the chocolate melts into the cream
2. Take the bowl off the heat and whisk the cocoa powder, stevia, rum and salt into the mixture until smooth and silky
3. Give it a taste...add more rum, salt and sweetener to suit your taste preferences!
4. Pour into a pouring jug and store in the fridge until required

Nutrition Info: Calories: 313;Fat: 28 grams ;Protein: 3 grams ;Total carbs: 10 grams ;Net carbs: 6 grams

Low-carb Macadamia Nut Brownies

Servings: 4-5

Cooking Time: 20 Minutes

Ingredients:

- 6 tablespoons almond flour
- 6 tablespoons chopped macadamia nuts
- 2 ½ tablespoons salted butter
- 1 large egg
- ½ teaspoon vanilla extract
- 6 tablespoons erythritol
- 2 tablespoons coconut oil
- 1 ½ tablespoons cocoa powder
- ¾ teaspoon baking powder
- ½ teaspoon instant coffee

Directions:

1. Line a small rimmed baking sheet or baking dish with parchment paper.
2. Add butter, coconut oil and erythritol into a mixing bowl. Beat with an electric hand mixer until creamy.
3. Add eggs and beat well.
4. Add all the dry ingredients except nuts and mix well. Add vanilla and half the nuts and stir well.
5. Pour the batter into the baking sheet. Spread it evenly.

6. Bake in a preheated oven 350° F for about 1– 20 minutes or until a toothpick when inserted in the middle comes out clean.

7. Remove from the oven. Let it cool on a wire rack for 15 minutes.

8. Cut into 4-5 equal pieces and serve.

Nutrition Info: Per Servings: Calories: 266 kcal, Fat: 31.3 g, Carbohydrates: 3.5 g, Protein: 5.6 g

Dairy-free Coconut Vanilla Pie

Servings: 8

Cooking Time:15 Minutes

Ingredients:

- 1 cup finely chopped toasted almonds
- ½ cup coconut flour
- ½ cup coconut oil
- 2 tsp gelatin
- ⅓ cup boiling water
- 2 cups full fat coconut cream
- 1 Tbsp vanilla extract
- 1 ½ tsp Stevia/your preferred keto sweetener

Directions:

1. Grease a pie pan with coconut oil and set aside
2. Combine the chopped almonds, coconut flour and coconut oil until it resembles wet sand
3. Press the almond/coconut oil mixture into your prepared pie pan
4. Pour the boiling water over the gelatin in a small bowl and stir until the gelatin dissolves into the water, leave to cool
5. In a large bowl, whip the coconut cream, vanilla and sweetener until thick and fluffy

6. Stir the cold gelatin water into the coconut cream mixture and pour the mixture into the pie dish on top of your nutty base

7. Place the pie into the fridge to chill and set for at least five hours, or overnight

8. Slice, serve, enjoy!

Nutrition Info: Calories: 36Fat: 35 grams ;Protein: 5 grams ;Total carbs: 9 grams ;Net carbs: 4 grams

Walnut-fruit Cake

Servings: 6

Cooking Time: 20 Minutes

Ingredients:

- 1/2 Cup of almond butter (softened)
- ¼ Cup of so Nourished granulated erythritol
- 1 Tablespoon of ground cinnamon
- ½ Teaspoon of ground nutmeg
- ¼ Teaspoon of ground cloves
- 4 Large pastured eggs
- 1 Teaspoon of vanilla extract
- ½ Teaspoon of almond extract
- 2 Cups of almond flour
- ½ Cup of chopped walnuts
- ¼ Cup of dried of unsweetened cranberries
- ¼ Cup of seedless raisins

Directions:

1. Preheat your oven to a temperature of about 350 F and grease an 8-inch baking tin of round shape with coconut oil.
2. Beat the granulated erythritol on a high speed until it becomes fluffy.
3. Add the cinnamon, the nutmeg, and the cloves; then blend your ingredients until they become smooth.

4. Crack in the eggs and beat very well by adding one at a time, plus the almond extract and the vanilla.
5. Whisk in the almond flour until it forms a smooth batter then fold in the nuts and the fruit.
6. Spread your mixture into your prepared baking pan and bake it for about 20 minutes.
7. Remove the cake from the oven and let cool for about 5 minutes.
8. Dust the cake with the powdered erythritol.
9. Serve and enjoy your cake!

Nutrition Info: Calories: 250;Fat: 11g;Carbohydrates: 12g;Fiber: 2g;Protein: 7g

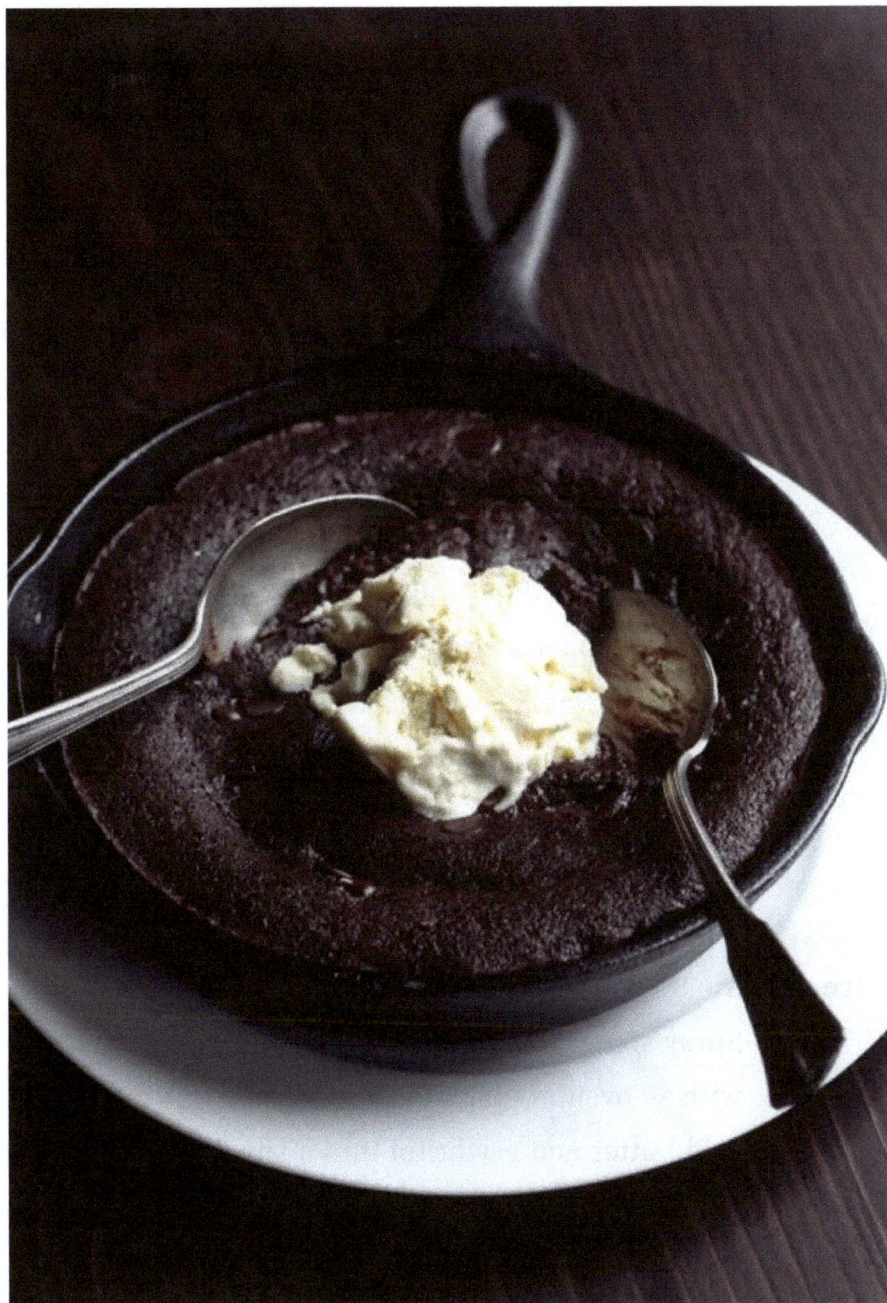

Keto Skillet Brownies

Servings: 8

Cooking Time: 30 Minutes

Ingredients:

- For brownies:
- ¾ cup butter
- 2/3 cup cocoa powder, unsweetened
- 2 eggs, at room temperature
- 2/3 cup erythritol
- ¼ teaspoon salt
- ½ cup almond flour
- ½ cup chopped walnuts
- 1 teaspoon vanilla extract
- 1 teaspoon baking powder
- For peanut butter drizzle:
- 2 tablespoons butter
- 2 tablespoons peanut butter

Directions:

1. Spray some cooking spray on a -inch cast iron skillet with an ovenproof handle.
2. Add butter and erythritol into a small pan. Place the pan over low heat and stir until erythritol dissolves completely. Transfer into a mixing bowl.

3. Add eggs into a mixing bowl and beat well. Next beat in almond flour and baking powder.

4. Add walnuts and fold gently.

5. Pour batter into the skillet and spread it evenly.

6. Bake in a preheated oven 350° F for about 25 – 30 minutes or until it just sets in the middle. If you insert a toothpick, you should have a bit of the batter sticking to it.

7. Remove from the oven and let it cool on a wire rack for a while.

8. Meanwhile make the peanut butter drizzle by adding butter and peanut butter into a microwave safe bowl. Microwave on high for about a minute or so until the mixture melts. Stir every 20 seconds.

9. Cut into 8 equal pieces and place in bowls. Drizzle peanut butter drizzle on the brownies and serve.

10. Store leftover brownies in a Ziploc bag. Seal and chill until use. These can keep for a week. Store the leftover drizzle in a small microwave safe container and refrigerate until use. Melt in the microwave and drizzle over the brownies and serve.

Nutrition Info: Per Servings: Calories: 364 kcal, Fat: 48.3 g, Carbohydrates: 5.8 g, Protein: 8.5 g

Chocolate Avocado Brownies

Servings: 24

Cooking Time: 35 Minutes

Ingredients:

- For dry ingredients:
- 6 ounces blanched almond flour
- 2 teaspoons baking powder
- ½ teaspoon baking soda
- ½ cup erythritol
- ½ teaspoon salt
- 2 teaspoons stevia powder
- For wet ingredients:
- 2 cups mashed avocados
- ½ cup cocoa powder
- 6 tablespoons refined coconut oil
- 7 ounces stevia sweetened dark chocolate, melted
- 1 teaspoon vanilla extract
- 4 eggs

Directions:

1. Add avocados into a food processor bowl. Pulse until creamy.
2. Add all the other wet ingredients, one at a time and process each time until well combined.

3. Add all the dry ingredients into a bowl and stir. Transfer into the food processor and pulse until well incorporated.

4. Line a large baking dish (9 x 13 inches) with parchment paper. Pour batter into the dish.

5. Bake in a preheated oven at 3° F for about 35 minutes or until a toothpick when inserted in the center comes out with a few particles of the brownie stuck on it.

6. Remove from the oven and cool on a rack. Cut into 24 pieces.

7. Store leftovers in an airtight container in the refrigerator for 6-days or frozen for a month.

Nutrition Info: Per Servings: Calories: 116 kcal, Fat: 10 g, Carbohydrates: 5 g, Protein: 3 g

Ricotta Parfait Cups

Servings: 5

Cooking Time:10 Minutes

Ingredients:

- 13 oz full fat ricotta cheese
- 3 oz full fat mascarpone cheese
- ¾ tsp Stevia/you preferred keto sweetener
- 1 tsp vanilla extract
- 1 cup mixed berries (strawberries, blueberries and raspberries)
- ¼ cup chopped walnuts
- ¼ cup chopped almonds
- ¾ cup heavy cream

Directions:

1. Stir together the ricotta, mascarpone, sweetener and vanilla until smooth and combined
2. Spoon half of the ricotta mixture into four dessert dishes
3. Scatter the berries over the ricotta mixture
4. Spoon the rest of the ricotta mixture over the berries and finish by scattering the toasted nuts over the top
5. Pop the parfaits into the fridge to chill for at least an hour
6. Serve!

Nutrition Info: Calories: 402;Fat: 36 grams ;Protein: 12 grams ;Total carbs: 8 grams ;Net carbs: grams

Classic Gluten Free Keto Blondies

Servings: 30-32

Cooking Time: 22 – 25 Minutes

Ingredients:

- 2 2/3 cups almond flour
- 1 teaspoon salt
- 1 cup butter
- 2 teaspoons vanilla extract
- 2 teaspoons baking powder
- 2 cups Swerve brown sugar substitute
- 2 eggs
- Optional:
- Chopped nuts or chocolate chips

Directions:

1. Take a large baking dish (9 x inches) and spray some cooking spray in it.
2. Add flour, salt and baking powder into a bowl and stir.
3. Add butter into a microwave safe bowl. Place in the microwave and cook on high for 40 – 50 seconds until butter melts.
4. Stir in the Swerve brown sugar. Whisk well.
5. Add vanilla and eggs and mix well.
6. Add the mixture of dry ingredients and mix well.
7. Fold in the optional add-in if using.

8. Spoon into the prepared baking dish.

9. Bake in a preheated oven 350° F for about 22-25 minutes. It should be almost set but not firm, or slightly undercooked.

10. Remove from the oven and let it cool on a wire rack.

11. Cut into 30-32 squares and serve.

12. Transfer leftovers into airtight container. Refrigerate until use. These can keep for 5-6 days.

Nutrition Info: Per Servings: Calories: 79 kcal, Fat: 8.3 g, Carbohydrates: 0.7 g, Protein: 1.1 g

Fresh Strawberry Sage Popsicles

Servings: 12

Cooking Time: 2 Minutes

Ingredients:

- 16 medium to large strawberries, hulled, chopped
- ¼ cup water
- 6 sage leaves

Directions:

1. Add strawberries, sage and water into a blender and blend until smooth.
2. Pour into Popsicle molds. Insert Popsicle sticks and freeze until firm.
3. To serve: Dip the Popsicle molds in a bowl of warm water for 15 – 20 seconds. The Popsicles will loosen up. Remove from the molds and serve.

Nutrition Info: per Servings: Calories: 5.3 kcal, Fat: 0.1 g, Carbohydrates: 1.2 g, Protein: 0.2 g

Dairy-free Frosted Coconut Lime Cupcakes

Servings: 12

Cooking Time:40 Minutes

Ingredients:

- 2 cups ground almonds
- 1 cup unsweetened dried coconut (the finely-chopped kind, not thread)
- 1 tsp Stevia/your preferred keto sweetener
- 1 tsp baking powder
- 3 eggs
- Juice and zest of 5 limes
- ½ cup coconut oil
- Frosting:
- 1 cup coconut cream
- ½ cup unsweetened coconut thread
- Juice and zest of 1 lime
- ½ tsp Stevia/your preferred keto sweetener

Directions:

1. Preheat the oven to 360 degrees Fahrenheit and line a -hole muffin pan with cupcake cases
2. In a large bowl, toss together the ground almonds, coconut, sweetener and baking powder

3. In a smaller bowl, beat together the eggs, lime juice and coconut oil

4. Fold the wet ingredients into the dry ingredients

5. Spoon the mixture into your prepared cupcake cases and pop the tray into the oven to bake for about 235 minutes or until just cooked. A skewer should come out clean

6. Leave the cupcakes to cool completely

7. Make the frosting: beat together the coconut cream, lime juice and sweetener until thick and fluffy

8. Spread the frosting over the cupcakes then sprinkle the coconut thread and lime zest over the top

9. Enjoy with a hot cup of coffee!

Nutrition Info: Calories: 299;Fat: 29 grams ;Protein: 6 grams ;Total carbs: 6 grams ;Net carbs: 3 grams

Butter Pecan Mascarpone And Ricotta Cream Cups

Servings: 6

Cooking Time:20 Minutes

Ingredients:

- 9 oz full fat mascarpone cheese
- 5 oz full fat ricotta cheese
- ⅓ cup heavy cream
- 2 tsp vanilla extract
- 1 tsp Stevia/your preferred keto sweetener
- 3 oz butter
- 1 ½ cups pecan nuts
- Pinch of sea salt
- Pinch of Stevia/your preferred keto sweetener

Directions:

1. Whip together the mascarpone, ricotta, cream, vanilla and sweetener until thick and fluffy
2. Place the butter into a frying pan over a medium-high heat and allow the butter to melt and become frothy
3. Add the pecan nuts and sweetener to the hot butter and stir as the nuts toast and become coated in butter. The nuts should be golden, fragrant and have a delicious toasted flavor when tasted

4. Leave the pecans to cool before folding them into the ricotta/mascarpone mixture
5. Spoon the mixture into dessert dishes and place into the fridge to chill for at least an hour before serving!

Nutrition Info: Calories: 580;Fat: grams ;Protein: 8 grams ;Total carbs: 6 grams ;Net carbs: 3 grams

Dairy-free Coffee Fudge Mug Cake

Servings: 2

Cooking Time:10 Minutes

Ingredients:

- ⅔ cup ground almonds
- 3 Tbsp unsweetened cocoa powder
- 1 tsp baking powder
- Pinch of salt
- 2 tsp espresso powder
- 6 Tbsp almond milk
- ½ tsp vanilla extract
- ½ tsp Stevia/your preferred keto sweetener

Directions:

1. Combine all ingredients in a small bowl and divide the mixture between two mugs
2. Place the mugs into the microwave and cook on high for 1 minute
3. Check the brownies and if they're still completely liquid then put them back in for second intervals until you reach the desired doneness. I like mine to be super gooey in the middle but cooked around the edges
4. Serve with coconut yogurt!

Nutrition Info: Calories: 217;Fat: 18 grams ;Protein: 8 grams ;Total carbs: 13 grams ;Net carbs: 6 grams

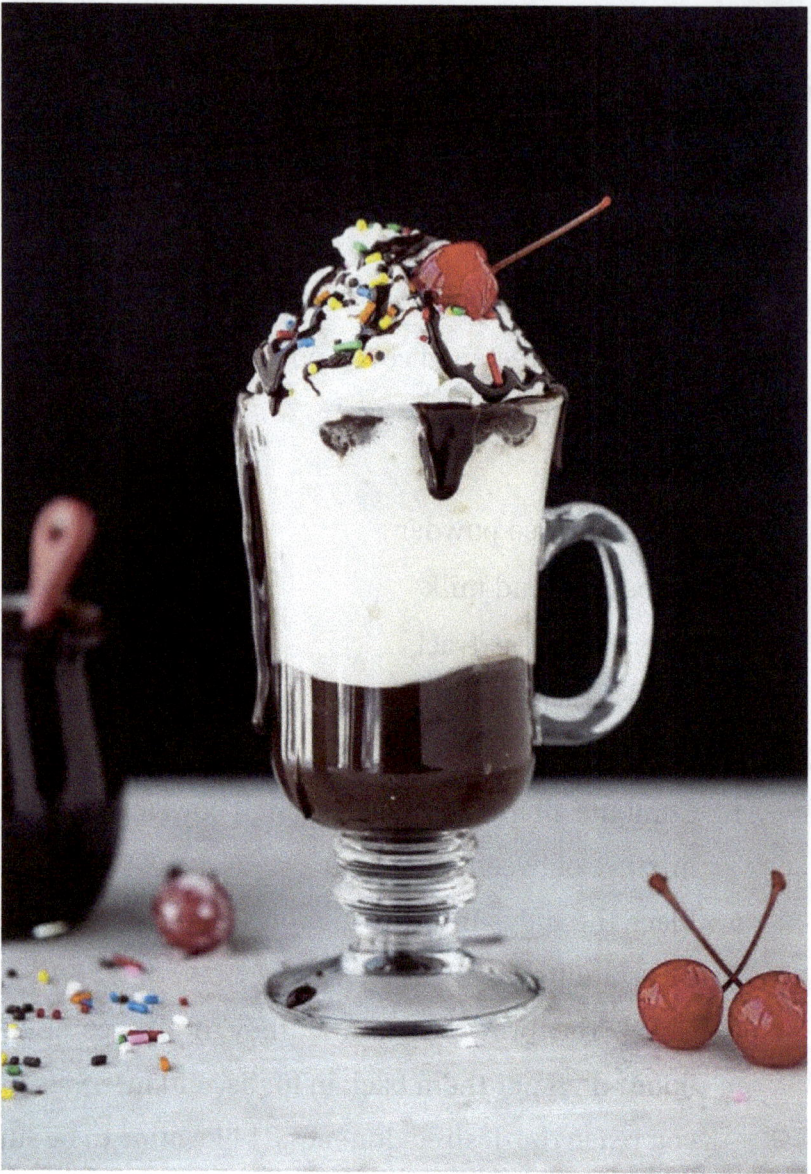

Raspberry Cake With White Chocolate Sauce

Servings:5-6

Cooking Time: 60 Minutes

Ingredients:

- 5 Ounces of melted cacao butter
- 2 Ounces of grass-fed ghee
- ½ Cup of coconut cream
- 1 Cup of green banana flour
- 3 Teaspoons of pure vanilla
- 4 Large eggs
- ½ Cup of as Lakanto Monk Fruit
- 1 Teaspoon of baking powder
- 2 Teaspoons of apple cider vinegar
- 2 Cup of raspberries
- For the white chocolate sauce:
- 3 and ½ ounces of cacao butter
- ½ Cup of coconut cream
- 2 Teaspoons of pure vanilla extract
- 1 Pinch of salt

Directions:

1. Preheat your oven to a temperature of about 280 degrees Fahrenheit.

2. Combine the green banana flour with the pure vanilla extract, the baking powder, the coconut cream, the eggs, the cider vinegar and the monk fruit and mix very well.

3. Leave the raspberries aside and line a cake loaf tin with a baking paper .

4. Pour in the batter into the baking tray and scatter the raspberries over the top of the cake.

5. Place the tray in your oven and bake it for about 60 minutes; in the meantime, prepare the sauce by

6. Combine the cacao cream, the vanilla extract, the cacao butter and the salt in a saucepan over a low heat.

7. Mix all your ingredients with a fork to make sure the cacao butter mixes very well with the cream.

8. Remove from the heat and set aside to cool a little bit; but don't let it harden.

9. Drizzle with the chocolate sauce.

10. Scatter the cake with more raspberries.

11. Slice your cake; then serve and enjoy it!

Nutrition Info: Calories: 323;Fat: 31.5g;Carbohydrates: 9.9g;Fiber: 4g;Protein: 5g

Lemon Curd

Servings: 6

Cooking Time:25 Minutes

Ingredients:

- 4 oz butter
- 1 tsp Stevia/your preferred keto sweetener
- Juice and zest of 5 lemons
- 3 whole eggs
- 2 egg yolks

Directions:

1. Place a heatproof bowl over a saucepan of simmering water
2. Add the butter, sweetener, lemon zest and juice to the bowl and stir as the butter melts
3. Whisk as you add the eggs and egg yolks to the bowl and keep whisking as the curd thickens (it should be able to coat the back of a spoon)
4. Pour the curd into sterilized jars or pouring jugs and store in the fridge until needed

Nutrition Info: Calories: 198;Fat: 19 grams ;Protein: 4 grams ;Total carbs: 4 grams ;Net carbs: 4 grams

Keto Maple Pecan Blondies

Servings: 16

Cooking Time: 35 Minutes

Ingredients:

- ½ cup coconut flour
- 2 cups almond flour
- 1 ½ cups chopped walnuts
- 1 cup butter, melted (measure first and then melt)
- 2 teaspoons maple extract
- 4 teaspoons baking powder
- 1 cup Swerve
- 6 eggs

Directions:

1. Take a large baking dish (9 x inches). Take a large sheet of foil and place it in the dish so that it is hanging over a little bit over the edges of the dish.
2. Spray the foil with cooking spray.
3. Add Swerve and butter into a mixing bowl. Beat with an electric mixer until smooth.
4. Add eggs and maple extract and beat well.
5. Stir in the flours and baking powder. Add nuts and mix well.
6. Spoon the batter into the baking dish.
7. Bake in a preheated oven 350° F for about 35 minutes.

8. Remove from the oven and let it cool on a wire rack for a while. Place the baking dish in the refrigerator for a couple of hours.

9. Cut into 16 squares and serve.

10. Transfer leftovers into airtight container. Refrigerate until use. These can keep for 5-6 days.

Nutrition Info: Per Servings: Calories: 261.3 kcal, Fat: 24.6 g, Carbohydrates: 5.3 g, Protein: 6.6 g

Dairy-free Butterscotch Fudge Balls

Servings: 12

Cooking Time:10 Minutes

Ingredients:

- 1 cup raw cashews
- ½ cup coconut cream
- 1 tsp Stevia/your preferred keto sweetener
- 1 ½ tsp sea salt
- 3 tsp butterscotch or caramel essence
- 2 Tbsp coconut oil
- 2 tsp vanilla extract
- 1 cup ground almonds

Directions:

1. Line a baking tray with baking paper and set aside
2. Place the cashews, coconut cream, sweetener, sea salt, butterscotch, coconut oil and vanilla into a food processor and blitz until super smooth and creamy
3. Transfer the mixture into a bowl and stir in the ground almonds to create a thick, paste-like consistency
4. Roll the mixture into balls and place onto your prepared tray
5. Place the tray into the fridge to set and firm up for at least an hour
6. Store in an airtight container in the fridge!

Nutrition Info: Calories: 13;Fat: 12 grams ;Protein: 3 grams ;Total carbs: 5 grams ;Net carbs: 4 grams

Creamy Keto Turmeric Popsicles

Servings: 8

Cooking Time: 5 Minutes

Ingredients:

- 2 cups coconut milk
- 2 teaspoon ground ginger
- Stevia or erythritol to taste
- 1 tablespoon turmeric powder
- A pinch pepper

Directions:

1. Add coconut milk, ginger, erythritol, turmeric powder and pepper into a small pan. Place the pan over medium heat. Stir frequently until the sweetener is dissolved. Turn off the heat and let cool to room temperature.

2. Divide into 8 Popsicle molds. Insert the popsicle sticks and freeze until firm.

3. To serve: Dip the Popsicle molds in a bowl of warm water for 15 – 20 seconds. The Popsicles will loosen up. Remove from the molds and serve.

Nutrition Info: per Servings: Calories: 11.3 kcal, Fat: 1.1 g, Carbohydrates: 0.3 g, Protein: 0 g

Collagen Protein Brownies

Servings: 8

Cooking Time: 15-18 Minutes

Ingredients:

- For dry ingredients:
- 6 scoops unflavored collagen peptides
- ¼ cup unsweetened cocoa powder
- ¼ teaspoon baking soda
- 6 tablespoons stevia-erythritol blend
- 6 tablespoons almond flour
- ¼ teaspoon salt (optional)
- For wet ingredients:
- 2 large egg whites
- 1 teaspoon vanilla extract (optional)
- ¼ cup creamy almond butter
- 2 tablespoons unsweetened almond milk
- 1 ounce dark chocolate chips

Directions:

1. Add all the dry ingredients into a mixing bowl and stir.
2. Add all the other ingredients except chocolate chips into the bowl of dry ingredients and mix until well combined.
3. Add chocolate chips and stir.

4. Place a sheet of parchment paper in a 6 x 6 inch baking dish.

5. Bake in a preheated oven 3° F for about 15 – 16 minutes or until it just sets in the middle. If you insert a toothpick, you should have a bit of the batter sticking to it.

6. Remove from the oven. Let cool on a wire rack completely.

7. Cut into 8 equal pieces and serve.

8. Store leftovers in an airtight container in the refrigerator for 6-7 days or frozen for a month.

Nutrition Info: Per Servings: Calories: 156 kcal, Fat: g, Carbohydrates: 6 g, Protein: 5.6 g

Keto Tiramisu

Servings: 8

Cooking Time:1 Hour

Ingredients:

- Biscuits:
- 3 oz butter, melted
- 1 egg
- ¼ tsp almond essence
- 1 tsp vanilla extract
- 1 cup ground almonds
- ½ cup slivered almonds, toasted
- ½ tsp Stevia/your preferred keto sweetener
- 1 tsp baking powder
- ¼ cup very strong espresso mixed with a tiny pinch of Stevia/your preferred keto sweetener
- 1 lb mascarpone cheese
- 1 Tbsp Marsala wine
- 1 tsp Stevia/your preferred keto sweetener
- To top the tiramisu:
- 1 cup heavy cream
- ½ tsp Stevia/your preferred keto sweetener
- 2 Tbsp unsweetened cocoa powder

Directions:

1. Preheat the oven to 360 degrees Fahrenheit and line a tray with baking paper

2. Whisk together the melted butter, egg, almond essence and vanilla extract

3. Stir the ground almonds, slivered almonds, sweetener and baking powder into the wet ingredients until thoroughly combined

4. Roll the dough into balls, place onto the lined tray and press down with your hand or a fork. Place the tray into the oven and bake for about 20 minutes or until the cookies are golden. Leave the cookies to cool completely

5. Crush the cooled biscuits and scatter them into a rectangular dish, pour the coffee over top and leave it to soak in

6. Stir together the mascarpone, sweetener and Marsala wine

7. Spoon the mascarpone mixture over the coffee-soaked biscuits

8. Whip the cream with the sweetener until soft and fluffy, spoon over the mascarpone

9. Sift the cocoa over the cream before serving!

Nutrition Info: Calories: 452;Fat: 45 grams ;Protein: 7 grams ;Total carbs: 8 grams ;Net carbs: 5 grams

Pistachio Ricotta Cakes With Mascarpone Frosting

Servings: 12

Cooking Time:45 Minutes

Ingredients:

- 2 cups ground almonds
- ¾ cup crushed pistachios
- 1 tsp baking powder
- 1 ½ tsp Stevia/your preferred keto sweetener
- 2 tsp vanilla extract
- 4 eggs
- 9 oz full fat ricotta cheese
- Frosting:
- 9 oz full fat mascarpone
- ½ tsp Stevia/your preferred keto sweetener
- ½ cup crushed pistachios

Directions:

1. Preheat the oven to 360 degrees Fahrenheit and grease a -hole muffin pan with butter
2. Stir together the ground almonds, pistachios, baking powder and sweetener
3. In a separate bowl, beat the vanilla, eggs and ricotta cheese until smooth

4. Fold the egg mixture into the dry ingredients until just combined

5. Spoon the batter into your prepared muffin pan and place it into the oven to bake for3minutes or until the cakes bounce back when touched

6. Make the frosting: stir together the mascarpone, sweetener and pistachios

7. Leave the cakes to cool completely before slathering with frosting!

Nutrition Info: Calories: 30Fat: 27 grams ;Protein: 11 grams ;Total carbs: 8 grams ;Net carbs: 5 grams

Berry Coulis

Servings: 5

Cooking Time:15 Minutes

Ingredients:

- ½ cup frozen strawberries
- ½ cup frozen raspberries
- ½ cup frozen blueberries
- 1 tsp Stevia/your preferred keto sweetener
- Juice of 1 lemon
- 3 Tbsp avocado oil

Directions:

1. Place all ingredients into a food processor and blitz until very smooth
2. Transfer the coulis into a sieve and place it over a bowl
3. Use a spatula to press the coulis through the sieve and into the bowl below, this will leave the berry seeds in the sieve, and will create a super smooth coulis
4. Discard the seeds in the sieve and transfer the coulis to a pouring jug and store in the fridge until needed

Nutrition Info: Calories: 96;Fat: 8 grams;Protein: 0 grams ;Total carbs: 7 grams ;Net carbs: grams

Chocolate And Strawberry Ice Cream Bars

Servings: 10

Cooking Time:10 Minutes

Ingredients:

- 2 avocados, flesh scooped out
- 2 cups heavy cream
- 3 Tbsp cocoa powder
- 1 tsp Stevia/your preferred keto sweetener
- 1 cup chopped fresh strawberries

Directions:

1. Place the avocado flesh in a food processor and blitz until super smooth and creamy
2. With an electric egg beater, whip the cream, cocoa powder and stevia until thick, soft and fluffy
3. Fold the smooth avocado into the cream mixture then fold the strawberries through
4. Spoon the mixture into your popsicle molds, put the lids on and place into the freezer overnight
5. Leave the bars in the molds at room temperature for a few minutes before sliding them out and enjoying in the sun!

Nutrition Info: Calories: 220;Fat: 22 grams;Protein: 2 grams;Total carbs: grams ;Net carbs: 3 grams

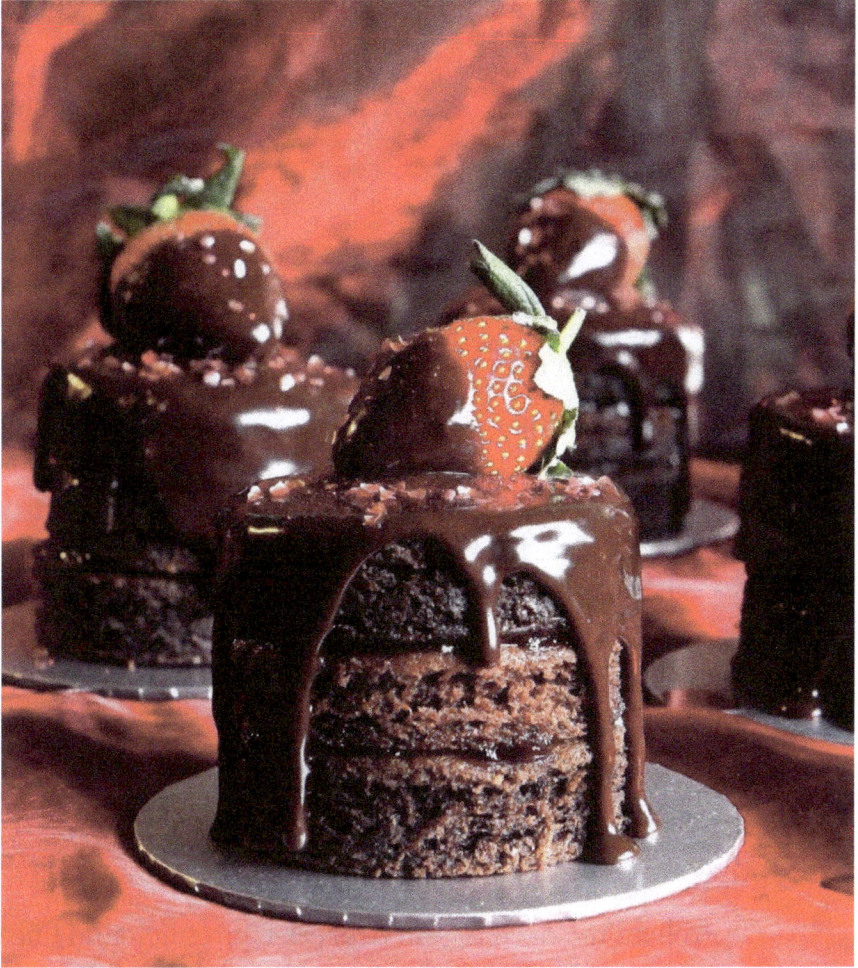

Dairy-free Lemon Drizzle Cake

Servings: 10

Cooking Time:50 Minutes

Ingredients:

- 3 eggs, separated
- ½ cup fresh lemon juice
- Zest of 3 lemons
- ½ cup coconut oil
- 2 tsp Stevia/your preferred keto sweetener
- 1 tsp baking powder
- 2 cups ground almonds
- Drizzle:
- ½ cup fresh lemon juice
- 1 tsp Stevia/your preferred keto sweetener

Directions:

1. Preheat the oven to 360 degrees Fahrenheit and line a cake pan with baking paper
2. In a large bowl, beat the egg whites with electric egg beaters until very stiff
3. Whisk together the egg yolks, sweetener, lemon juice, lemon zest and coconut oil
4. Toss together the ground almonds and the baking powder

5. Take a little bit of your beaten egg whites and fold them into the egg/lemon mixture, then fold in a little bit of the ground almonds. Repeat this until all of the ingredients are combined. Be very gentle so you don't knock the air out of your egg whites! The air will help the cake to rise

6. Pour the batter into your prepared cake pan and pop it into your preheated oven to bake for about 30-40 minutes or until a skewer comes out clean

7. As the cake is baking, prepare the drizzle: place the lemon juice and sweetener into a saucepan with a dash of water and bring to a simmer. Simmer until the mixture is sticky and a little thicker than before

8. As soon as you take the cake out of the oven, pour the drizzle over the top and leave to soak in!

9. Serve warm, with a dollop of coconut yogurt

Nutrition Info: Calories: 236;Fat: 22 grams;Protein: 6 grams ;Total carbs: 6 grams ;Net carbs: 3 grams

Raspberry Crumble

Servings: 5

Cooking Time:35 Minutes

Ingredients:

- 2 cups raspberries (fresh or frozen)
- 1 cup ground almonds
- ½ cup dried unsweetened coconut
- 4 oz butter, cold
- 2 tsp Stevia/your preferred keto sweetener
- Pinch of salt
- 1 tsp ground cinnamon
- ½ cup slivered almonds

Directions:

1. Preheat the oven to 360 degrees Fahrenheit and have a small baking dish waiting by
2. Place the raspberries into the bottom of the dish and set aside
3. Place the ground almonds, coconut, butter, stevia, salt and cinnamon into a food processor and pulse until it resembles a crumbly, sandy texture with a few larger butter chunks (pea-sized)
4. Sprinkle the crumble over the raspberries
5. Sprinkle the slivered almonds over the crumble

6. Place the crumble into the oven and bake for about 25 minutes or until the crumble is nice and golden!

7. Serve with plenty of heavy cream

Nutrition Info: Calories: 395;Fat: 37 grams;Protein: 7 grams;Total carbs: 14 grams ;Net carbs: 6 grams

Gooey Chocolate Brownies

Servings: 16

Cooking Time:40 Minutes

Ingredients:

- 5 oz 72% cocoa dark chocolate
- 5 oz butter
- 3 eggs
- 2 tsp vanilla extract (pure, unsweetened)
- 1 cup ground almonds
- 3 Tbsp unsweetened cocoa powder
- 1 tsp Stevia/your preferred keto sweetener
- 1 heaping tsp sea salt

Directions:

1. Preheat the oven to 360 degrees Fahrenheit and line a brownie pan with baking paper
2. Place the chocolate and butter into a heatproof bowl and place over a pot of simmering water. Stir as the butter and chocolate melt together. Remove from the heat and set aside to cool
3. Add the eggs and vanilla to the melted chocolate and butter mixture and whisk until thoroughly combined
4. Stir the ground almonds, cocoa, sweetener and salt into the chocolate mixture until smooth and combined

5. Spread the batter into your prepared pan and place into the oven to bake for about 20-30 minutes depending on your oven and your preferred doneness. I like my brownies to be gooey so I only cooked mine for 20 minutes!

6. Leave to cool slightly before cutting into squares and serving

7. Freeze any leftovers and have them on hand for your next chocolate craving

Nutrition Info: Calories: 14Fat: 12.9 grams ;Protein: 3.3 grams ;Total carbs: 7.3 grams ;Net carbs: 4.9 grams

Ketogenic Orange Cake

Servings: 8

Cooking Time: 50minutes

Ingredients:

- 2 and ½ cups of almond flour
- 2 Unwaxed washed oranges
- 5 Large separated eggs
- 1 Teaspoon of baking powder
- 2 Teaspoons of orange extract
- 1 Teaspoon of vanilla bean powder
- 6 Seeds of cardamom pods crushed
- 16 drops of liquid stevia; about 3 teaspoons
- 1 Handful of flaked almonds to decorate

Directions:

1. Preheat your oven to a temperature of about 350 Fahrenheit.
2. Line a rectangular bread baking tray with a parchment paper.
3. Place the oranges into a pan filled with cold water and cover it with a lid.
4. Bring the saucepan to a boil, then let simmer for about 1 hour and make sure the oranges are totally submerged.

5. Make sure the oranges are always submerged to remove any taste of bitterness.

6. Cut the oranges into halves; then remove any seeds; and drain the water and set the oranges aside to cool down.

7. Cut the oranges in half and remove any seeds, then puree it with a blender or a food processor.

8. Separate the eggs; then whisk the egg whites until you see stiff peaks forming.

9. Add all your ingredients except for the egg whites to the orange mixture and add in the egg whites; then mix.

10. Pour the batter into the cake tin and sprinkle with the flaked almonds right on top.

11. Bake your cake for about 50 minutes.

12. Remove the cake from the oven and set aside to cool for 5 minutes.

13. Slice your cake; then serve and enjoy its incredible taste!

Nutrition Info: Calories: 164;Fat: 12g;Carbohydrates: 7.1;Fiber: 2.7g;Protein: 10.9g

Strawberry Shortcakes

Servings: 12

Cooking Time:35 Minutes

Ingredients:

- 3 cups ground almonds
- 1 ½ tsp Stevia/your preferred keto sweetener
- Pinch of salt
- 1 tsp baking powder
- 3 eggs
- 1 cup heavy cream
- 2 tsp vanilla extract
- Few drops of pink food coloring (optional)
- 1 cup sliced fresh strawberries
- 1 cup heavy cream
- 2 tsp Stevia/your preferred keto sweetener

Directions:

1. Preheat the oven to 360 degrees Fahrenheit and line a -hole muffin pan with cupcake cases
2. In a large bowl, combine the ground almonds, sweetener, salt and baking powder
3. In a small bowl, whisk together the eggs, cream, vanilla and food coloring
4. Pour the wet ingredients into the dry ingredients and stir until just combined

5. Spoon the batter into your prepared cupcake cases and pop the tray into the oven to bake for about 2minutes or until the cakes are just set and a skewer comes out clean

6. Leave the cakes to cool completely

7. Whip the cream and stevia until the cream is soft and fluffy

8. Slice the cupcakes in half (so you have a top and bottom) and place a layer of strawberry slices onto the bottom half. Place a dollop of cream on top of the strawberries and place the top half of the cupcake on top of the cream

9. Serve right away so the cream stays fresh and fluffy!

Nutrition Info: Calories: 301;Fat: 28 grams ;Protein: 7 grams ;Total carbs: 8 grams;Net carbs: 5 grams

Mini Ginger Cheesecakes

Servings: 12

Cooking Time:45 Minutes

Ingredients:

- Base:
- 1 ½ cups ground almonds
- ½ cup roughly chopped walnuts
- 4 oz melted butter
- 1 tsp ground ginger
- Pinch of salt
- ½ tsp Stevia/your preferred keto sweetener
- Filling:
- 1 lb full fat cream cheese
- 9 oz full fat sour cream
- 3 eggs
- 2 tsp ground ginger
- 1 tsp Stevia/your preferred keto sweetener

Directions:

1. Preheat the oven to 360 degrees Fahrenheit and line a -hole muffin pan with cupcake cases
2. Combine all of the base ingredients until you achieve a sandy texture
3. Press the base mixture into the bottom of each cupcake case and set aside

4. In a large bowl, beat together all of the filling ingredients until smooth and combined

5. Spoon the filling into the cupcake cases on top of the nutty base

6. Place the tray into the oven and bake for about 30-40 minutes or until the cheesecakes are just set but still a little soft in the middle

7. Leave the cheesecakes to cool completely before eating with a dollop of whipped cream!

Nutrition Info: Calories: 321;Fat: 30 grams;Protein: grams;Total carbs: 5 grams ;Net carbs: 3 grams

Chocolate And Raspberry Cupcakes

Servings: 12

Cooking Time:30 Minutes

Ingredients:

- 4 oz butter
- 3 oz 72% cocoa dark chocolate
- 6 eggs
- 2 tsp vanilla extract
- 3 Tbsp cocoa powder
- 1 ½ tsp Stevia/your preferred keto sweetener
- 1 cup ground almonds
- 1 tsp baking powder
- Pinch of salt
- ½ cup heavy cream
- 1 cup raspberries
- Cream frosting:
- 1 cup heavy whipping cream
- 2 Tbsp cocoa powder
- 1 tsp Stevia/your preferred keto sweetener

Directions:

1. Preheat the oven to 360 degrees Fahrenheit and line a -hole muffin pan with cupcake cases

2. Place the butter and chocolate into a heatproof bowl and place over a saucepan of boiling water. Stir until the butter and chocolate have melted together

3. Remove the bowl from the heat and leave to cool for about 5 minutes

4. Add the eggs and vanilla to the cooled chocolate mixture and whisk until thoroughly combined and smooth

5. Sift the cocoa powder, stevia, ground almonds and salt into the chocolate mixture and fold them in until the ingredients are just combined, but don't overmix

6. Fold the cream and raspberries into the batter

7. Spoon the batter into the cupcake cases

8. Place the tray into the preheated oven and bake for about 20 minutes or until the cakes are just set but still a little gooey in the middle

9. Leave the cupcakes to cool completely

10. To create the cream frosting: use a whisk or electric egg beaters to whip the cream, cocoa powder and stevia together until fluffy and soft

11. Pipe or spoon the cream frosting over the cupcakes before serving

Nutrition Info: Calories: 306;Fat: 29 grams ;Protein: 7 grams ;Total carbs: 8 grams ;Net carbs: 4 grams

Chocolate Self-saucing Pudding

Servings: 6

Cooking Time:50 Minutes

Ingredients:

- 4 oz butter, melted
- ½ cup heavy cream
- 2 eggs, lightly beaten
- 1 cup ground almonds
- 3 Tbsp cocoa powder
- 1 ½ tsp Stevia/your preferred keto sweetener
- 1 tsp baking powder
- 1 tsp sea salt
- Sauce:
- 1 cup boiling water
- 3 Tbsp cocoa powder
- 3 tsp Stevia/your preferred keto sweetener

Directions:

1. Preheat the oven to 360 degrees Fahrenheit and grease a brownie pan or any rectangular baking dish with butter
2. Whisk together the melted butter, cream and eggs until combined

3. Sift the ground almonds, cocoa powder, sweetener, baking powder and salt into the wet ingredients and stir until combined

4. Spoon the batter into your prepared dish

5. Combine the cocoa powder and sweetener in a small cup and sprinkle over the batter

6. Pour the boiling water over the batter (carefully!)

7. Carefully place the dish into the oven and bake for about 25-30 minutes or until just cooked but still saucy and gooey

8. Serve hot or warm, with cream!

Nutrition Info: Calories: 332;Fat: 33 grams ;Protein: 7 grams ;Total carbs: grams ;Net carbs: 5 grams

Dairy-free Raspberry Mousse

Servings: 5

Cooking Time:30 Minutes

Ingredients:

- 1 tsp gelatin
- ½ cup water
- 1 tsp Stevia/your preferred keto sweetener
- 2 cups full-fat coconut cream
- 1 tsp vanilla extract
- 1 ½ cups fresh raspberries

Directions:

1. Place the water into a saucepan over a medium-high heat until it reaches a gentle simmer
2. Add the gelatin to the water and stir as it dissolves into the water. Take the pan off the heat and allow the gelatin mixture to cool
3. Place the coconut cream, sweetener and vanilla extract into a large bowl and whip with electric beaters until thick, soft and creamy
4. Keep beating as you pour the gelatin water into the whipped coconut cream until it's completely incorporated
5. Fold the raspberries into the mixture
6. Spoon the mousse into five glass dessert dishes

7. Place into the fridge for about an hour or until set

8. Serve and enjoy!

Nutrition Info: Calories: 253;Fat: 24 grams ;Protein: 3 grams ;Total carbs: 8 grams;Net carbs: 3 grams

Dairy-free Lemon Custard

Servings: 4

Cooking Time:30 Minutes

Ingredients:

- 2 cups unsweetened almond milk
- 4 egg yolks
- 1 tsp Stevia/your preferred keto sweetener
- ½ cup fresh lemon juice
- Zest of 1 lemon
- ½ tsp cornstarch dissolved in 2 tsp water

Directions:

1. Place all ingredients into a saucepan and whisk thoroughly to combine. Ensure the egg yolks are all totally incorporated into the liquids
2. Place the saucepan over a medium heat and keep stirring as the custard thickens. Don't leave the saucepan alone on the heat as you risk a burnt custard!
3. Pour the custard into a pouring jug or bottle and store in the fridge until required
4. Serve anyway you like!

Nutrition Info: Calories: 83;Fat: 6 grams ;Protein: 4 grams ;Total carbs: 3 grams ;Net carbs: 2 grams

Salted Chocolate Mascarpone Whip

Servings: 4

Cooking Time:15 Minutes

Ingredients:

- ¾ cup heavy cream
- 9 oz full fat mascarpone cheese
- 3 Tbsp unsweetened cocoa powder
- 2 tsp vanilla extract
- 1 tsp Stevia/your preferred keto sweetener
- ½ tsp sea salt

Directions:

1. Whip the cream until soft and fluffy
2. Add the rest of the ingredients to the whipped cream and stir until combined and smooth
3. Spoon the whip into four dessert dishes and place into the fridge to chill for at least an hour
4. Serve with a little sprinkle of cocoa powder on top!

Nutrition Info: Calories: 467;Fat: 48 grams ;Protein: 6 grams ;Total carbs: 6 grams ;Net carbs: grams

Mocha Cake

Servings: 12

Cooking Time:45 Minutes

Ingredients:

- 7 oz butter, softened
- 2 tsp Stevia/your preferred keto sweetener
- 4 eggs
- 2 tsp vanilla extract
- 2 Tbsp instant espresso powder, dissolved in 1 Tbsp water
- 2 Tbsp cocoa powder
- 1 ½ cups ground almonds
- 2 tsp baking powder
- Pinch of salt
- Frosting:
- 8 oz full-fat plain cream cheese
- 4 oz butter, softened
- 3 tsp Stevia/your preferred keto sweetener
- 2 tsp espresso powder, dissolved in 2 tsp hot water

Directions:

1. Preheat the oven to 360 degrees Fahrenheit and line a cake pan with baking paper
2. Beat the butter, sweetener, eggs and vanilla extract with electric beaters until soft, creamy and fluffy

3. Add the coffee mixture, cocoa powder, ground almonds, baking powder and salt, stir until just combined
4. Pour the batter into your prepared cake pan and bake in your preheated oven for about 30-35 minutes or until a skewer comes out clean
5. Leave the cake to cool completely
6. Make the frosting: using an electric egg beater, beat together the cream cheese and butter until combined and creamy. Add the stevia and espresso mixture and beat until thoroughly combined
7. Spread the frosting over the cooled cake
8. Slice and serve with a cup of hot coffee!

Nutrition Info: Calories: 464;Fat: 45 grams ;Protein: 10 grams;Total carbs: grams ;Net carbs: 5 grams

Mint-choc Chip Whip

Servings: 5

Cooking Time:10 Minutes

Ingredients:

- 1 cup heavy whipping cream (1 cup before whipping)
- 1 tsp Stevia/your preferred keto sweetener
- Pinch of salt
- 1 or 2 drops of green food coloring (optional)
- ½ cup fresh mint leaves, finely chopped
- Few drops of peppermint essence (optional, but it gives a more minty flavor)
- 1 ½ oz 72% cocoa dark chocolate chips

Directions:

1. Place the cream, sweetener, salt, food coloring, mint and peppermint extract into a large bowl and use an electric egg beater to whip until the cream is thick and soft
2. Fold the chocolate chips into the cream mixture
3. Spoon the mixture into five dessert dishes and place into the fridge to chill for at least 2 hours
4. Serve with a fresh mint leaf!

Nutrition Info: Calories: 213;Fat: 20.2 grams ;Protein: 1.grams ;Total carbs: 6.3 grams ;Net carbs: 5.5 grams

Skillet Keto Blondie

Servings: 16

Cooking Time: 20 Minutes

Ingredients:

- For dry ingredients:
- ½ cup coconut flour
- 2/3 cups erythritol
- ½ teaspoon Himalayan pink salt
- For wet ingredients:
- 4 large eggs
- 4 ounces cacao butter
- 1 teaspoon almond extract (optional)
- 2 teaspoons vanilla extract
- 1 ½ cups almond butter
- 40 drops liquid stevia
- Other ingredients:
- 4 ounces baker's chocolate
- 2/3 cup shredded coconut

Directions:

1. Spray some cooking spray on a -inch cast iron skillet with an ovenproof handle.
2. Add all the dry ingredients into a bowl and stir.

3. Melt the cacao butter in a double boiler. Remove from the double boiler and transfer into a large mixing bowl. Let cool for a few minutes.

4. Add the rest of the wet ingredients into the mixing bowl (with cacao) and whisk well.

5. Add dry ingredients into the bowl of wet ingredients and mix until well incorporated.

6. Add coconut and chocolate and fold gently.

7. Pour the batter into the skillet and spread it evenly.

8. Bake in a preheated oven at 350° F for about 25 – 30 minutes or until light golden brown in color.

9. Remove from the oven and let it cool on a wire rack for a while.

10. Cut into 16 equal pieces and serve.

11. Store leftovers in a Ziploc bag. Seal it and chill until use. These can keep for a week.

Nutrition Info: Per Servings: Calories: 257.6 kcal, Fat: 28.8 g, Carbohydrates: 4.3 g, Protein: 8.1 g

Blueberry Mascarpone Pie

Servings: 10

Cooking Time:35 Minutes

Ingredients:

- 1 ½ cups ground almonds
- 4 oz butter, melted
- 1 egg, lightly beaten
- 1 tsp Stevia/your preferred keto sweetener
- Pinch of salt
- 3 cups blueberries (fresh or frozen)
- ½ tsp ground cinnamon
- 9 oz full-fat mascarpone cheese
- 1 tsp Stevia/your preferred keto sweetener
- 2 tsp vanilla extract

Directions:

1. Preheat the oven to 360 degrees Fahrenheit and grease a pie dish with butter
2. Combine the ground almonds, butter, egg, stevia and salt until thoroughly combined
3. Press the almond mixture into your prepared pie dish and place into the preheated oven to bake for 12 minutes
4. Place the blueberries into the prebaked pie crust and sprinkle the berries with cinnamon

5. Place the pie back into the oven and bake for about 10 minutes or until the blueberries are soft and juicy

6. With a fork, gently press the cooked blueberries to create a mushier, softer texture, leave to cool

7. Combine the mascarpone, sweetener and vanilla together until smooth and creamy

8. Spoon the mascarpone over the blueberries before serving!

Nutrition Info: Calories: 285;Fat: 26 grams;Protein: 5 grams;Total carbs: 11 grams ;Net carbs: 8 grams

Ketogenic Lava Cake

Servings: 2

Cooking Time: 10 Minutes

Ingredients:

- 2 Oz of dark chocolate; you should at least use chocolate of 85% cocoa solids
- 1 Tablespoon of super-fine almond flour
- 2 Oz of unsalted almond butter
- 2 Large eggs

Directions:

1. Heat your oven to a temperature of about 350 Fahrenheit.
2. Grease heat proof ramekins with almond butter.
3. Now, melt the chocolate and the almond butter and stir very well.
4. Beat the eggs very well with a mixer.
5. Add the eggs to the chocolate and the butter mixture and mix very well with almond flour and the swerve; then stir.
6. Pour the dough into 2 ramekins.
7. Bake for about 9 to 10 minutes.
8. Turn the cakes over plates and serve with pomegranate seeds!

Nutrition Info: Calories: 45Fat: 39g;Carbohydrates: 3.5g;Fiber: 0.8g;Protein: 11.7g

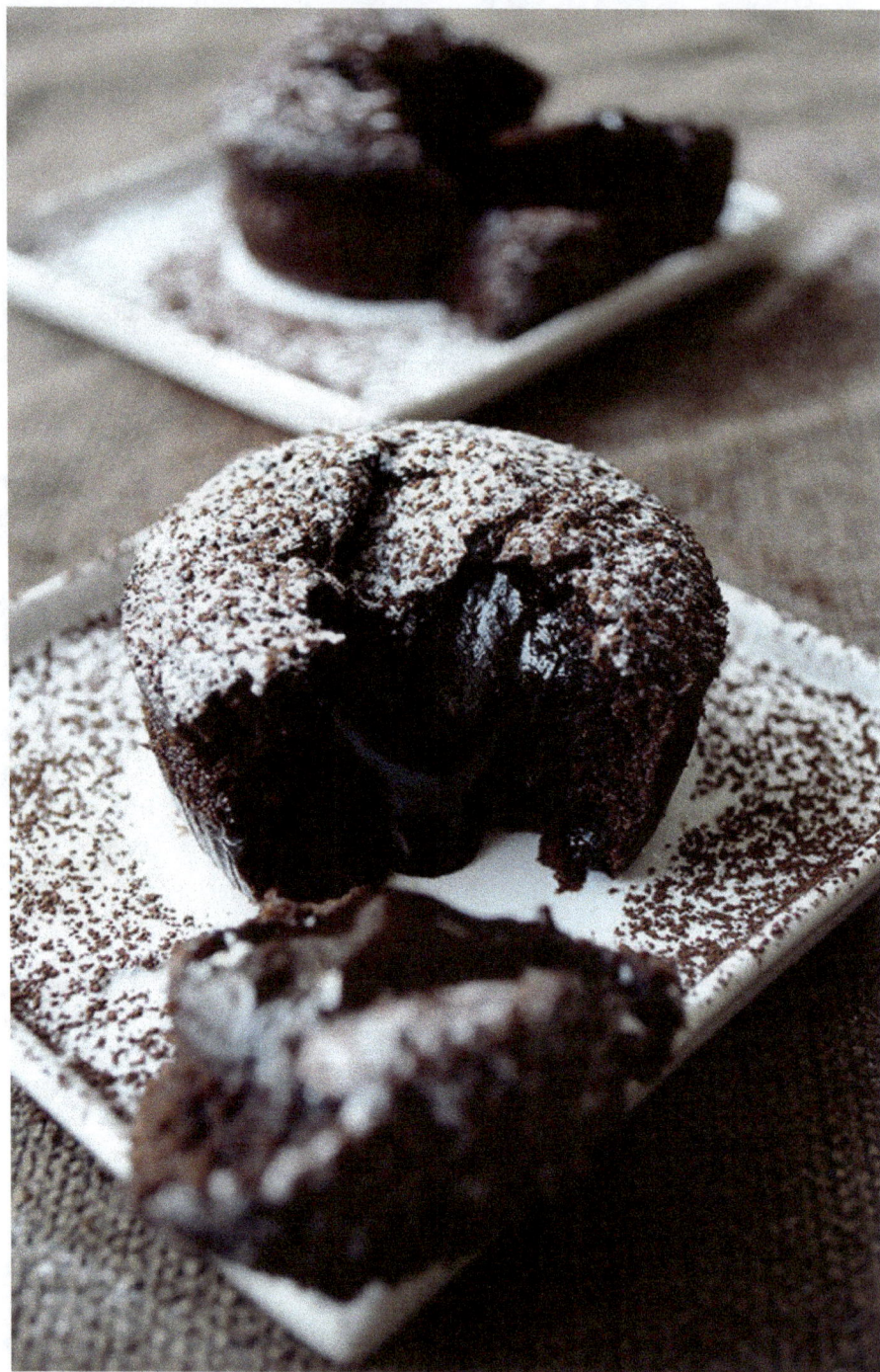

Almond Flour Blondies

Servings: 8

Cooking Time: 14-17 Minutes

Ingredients:

- 1 cup blanched almond flour
- 1 tablespoon coconut flour
- 3 tablespoons Swerve brown sugar substitute
- ½ teaspoon baking powder
- 2 tablespoons water
- 1/8 teaspoon fine sea salt

Directions:

1. Place a sheet of parchment paper in a baking dish (6 x 6 inches).
2. Add all the dry ingredients into a bowl and stir.
3. Stir in the water. Mix until well incorporated.
4. Pour batter into prepared baking dish.
5. Bake in a preheated oven 3° F for about 14 - 17 minutes. It should be almost set but not firm, slightly undercooked. Sprinkle flaky salt if using.
6. Remove from the oven and let it cool on a wire rack.
7. Cut into 8 equal squares and serve.
8. Transfer leftovers into airtight container. Refrigerate until use. These can keep for 5-6 days, or up to 6 months in the freezer.

Nutrition Info: Per Servings: Calories: 100 kcal, Fat: 7.1 g, Carbohydrates: 3.5 g, Protein: 3.1 g

Brownies With Almond Butter

Servings: 8

Cooking Time: 14 Minutes

Ingredients:

- ½ cup almond butter
- ¼ cup cocoa powder
- ¾ tablespoon coconut flour
- 2 large eggs
- 6 tablespoons granulated erythritol or Swerve
- A pinch of sea salt + extra pinch of salt if almond butter is unsalted

Directions:

1. Place rack in the lower third position in the oven. Place a sheet of parchment paper in a 6 x 6 inch baking dish.
2. Add almond butter and eggs into a mixing bowl. Beat with an electric hand mixer until smooth and well combined.
3. Add coconut flour, cocoa, sweetener and salt and beat until smooth. Let the batter rest for a couple of minutes.
4. Pour batter into the prepared baking dish.
5. Bake in a preheated oven 3° F for about 13 – 16 minutes or until it just sets in the middle. If you insert

a toothpick, you should have a bit of the batter sticking to it.

6. Remove from the oven. Let it cool on a wire rack completely.

7. Cut into 8 equal pieces and serve.

8. Leftovers can be stored in an airtight container in the refrigerator for 6-7 days or frozen for 2 months.

Nutrition Info: Per Servings: Calories: 153 kcal, Fat: 16.3 g, Carbohydrates: 4 g, Protein: 5 g

Keto Coconut Blondies

Servings: 16

Cooking Time: 20 Minutes

Ingredients:

- For dry ingredients:
- 1 cup coconut flour
- 2 teaspoons baking powder
- ½ cup unsweetened desiccated coconut
- ½ cup powdered Swerve or erythritol
- Shredded coconut, unsweetened, to garnish
- For wet ingredients:
- 2/3 cup melted coconut oil
- ½ cup coconut cream
- 4 teaspoons vanilla extract
- 6 large eggs

Directions:

1. Take a square baking dish (9 x 9 inches) and spray some cooking spray in it. Place a sheet of parchment paper in the dish.
2. Add all the wet ingredients into a large mixing bowl and whisk well.
3. Add all the dry ingredients into another bowl and stir. Transfer into the bowl of wet ingredients. Whisk until just incorporated and the mix is free of lumps.

4. Pour batter into prepared baking dish. Sprinkle shredded coconut on top of the mix.

5. Bake in a preheated oven 3° F for about 20 – 22 minutes. It should be almost set but not firm, or slightly undercooked.

6. Remove from the oven and let it cool on a wire rack.

7. Cut into 16 squares and serve.

8. Transfer leftovers into airtight container. Refrigerate until use. These can keep for 5-6 days.

Nutrition Info: Per Servings: Calories: 207 kcal, Fat: 18.6 g, Carbohydrates: 5.3 g, Protein: 4.1 g

Cream Cheese Frosting 3 Ways

Servings:12

Cooking Time:15 Minutes

Ingredients:

- Mint choc chip cream cheese frosting:
- 1 lb full fat cream cheese
- 6 oz butter softened
- 2 tsp Stevia/your preferred keto sweetener
- 4 oz 72% cocoa dark chocolate, finely chopped
- 1 tsp peppermint essence
- Couple of drops of green food coloring (optional)
- Mocha cream cheese frosting:
- 1 lb full fat cream cheese
- 6 oz butter softened
- 2 tsp Stevia/your preferred keto sweetener
- 2 Tbsp unsweetened cocoa powder
- 2 tsp instant espresso powder dissolved in 3 tsp water
- Lemon and raspberry cream cheese frosting:
- 1 lb full fat cream cheese
- 6 oz butter softened
- 2 tsp Stevia/your preferred keto sweetener
- ¾ cup raspberries
- Zest and juice of 1 lemon

Directions:

1. Beat together the cream cheese, butter and sweetener until soft and super creamy
2. Stir in your chosen flavorings until combined
3. Store in the fridge until required!

Nutrition Info: Mint choc chip cream cheese frosting:Calories: 291;Fat: 28 grams ;Protein: grams ;Total carbs: 4 grams ;Net carbs: 2 grams

Nutrition Info: Mocha cream cheese frosting:Calories: 237;Fat: 24 grams ;Protein: 3 grams ;Total carbs: 2 grams ;Net carbs: 2 grams

Nutrition Info: Lemon and raspberry cream cheese frosting :Calories: 240;Fat: 24 grams ;Protein: 3 grams ;Total carbs: 3 grams ;Net carbs: 2 grams

Keto Flourless Mocha Brownies

Servings: 24

Cooking Time: 40 Minutes

Ingredients:

- 12 ounces unsweetened Baker's chocolate
- 2 ½ cups monk fruit sweetener, divided
- 1 cup unsweetened cocoa powder
- 2 teaspoons pure vanilla extract
- ¾ cup coconut oil or unsalted butter
- 8 eggs, at room temperature, separated
- 4 tablespoons espresso powder
- 1 teaspoon salt

Directions:

1. Melt chocolate and coconut oil together in a double boiler.
2. When chocolate melts, lower heat to low. Add 1-cup monk fruit sweetener. Stir frequently until the sweetener melts. Turn off the heat. Remove the bowl from the double boiler and let it cool.
3. Beat the whites with an electric hand mixer set on high speed until stiff peaks are formed.
4. Add ½ cup monk fruit sweetener and set the speed to low. Beat until well combined and shiny.

5. Rinse the beater. Add remaining sweetener into the bowl of yolks and beat on high speed until well combined.

6. Add melted chocolate and fold gently with a rubber spatula.

7. Grease a large baking dish (9 x 13 inches) with cooking spray and line it with parchment paper.

8. Pour batter into the dish and spread evenly.

9. Bake in a preheated oven at 350° F for about 35 – 40 minutes or until a toothpick when inserted in the middle comes out clean.

10. Remove from the oven. Let it cool on a wire rack completely.

11. Cut into 8 equal pieces and serve.

12. Store leftovers in an airtight container in the refrigerator for 6-7 days or frozen for a month.

Nutrition Info: Per Servings: Calories: 148 kcal, Fat: 18 g, Carbohydrates: 6 g, Protein: 7 g

Mini Mixed Berry Cheesecake Muffins

Servings: 12

Cooking Time:35 Minutes

Ingredients:

- 2 cups ground almonds
- 1 tsp Stevia/your preferred keto sweetener
- 1 ½ tsp baking powder
- 3 eggs
- ½ cup cream
- 1 tsp vanilla extract
- Cheesecake topping:
- 9 oz full-fat, plain cream cheese
- 2 eggs
- 1 tsp Stevia/your preferred keto sweetener
- 1 ½ cups mixed berries (I use blueberries, strawberries and raspberries)

Directions:

1. Preheat the oven to 360 degrees Fahrenheit and line a -hole muffin pan with cupcake cases
2. In a large bowl, beat together the cream cheese, eggs and stevia until thick, soft and combined, set aside as you prep the muffin batter
3. Combine the ground almonds, sweetener and baking powder in a large bowl

4. In a small bowl, whisk together the eggs, cream and vanilla extract until combined

5. Gently fold the wet ingredients into the dry ingredients until just combined

6. Spoon the batter into the prepared cupcake cases

7. Sprinkle half of the berries over the muffin batter

8. Spoon the cheesecake mixture over the muffin batter and berries and place the rest of the berries over the cheesecake mixture

9. Place the pan into the oven and bake until the cheesecake portion is set and the muffin batter is cooked through, (stick a skewer into the cupcakes and there should only be cheesecake on the skewer when you take it out)

10. Leave to cool before devouring!

Nutrition Info: Calories: 2Fat: 18 grams ;Protein: 7 grams ;Total carbs: 6 grams ;Net carbs: 4 grams

Dairy-free Chocolate Cookies

Servings: 12

Cooking Time:25 Minutes

Ingredients:

- 3 Tbsp coconut oil (melted, if your coconut oil has solidified)
- 1 egg
- 1 tsp vanilla extract
- ⅓ cup almond milk
- 1 tsp Stevia/your preferred keto sweetener
- 2 cups ground almonds
- 1 tsp baking powder
- 5 oz 72% cocoa dark chocolate, roughly chopped
- Pinch of salt

Directions:

1. Preheat the oven to 360 degrees Fahrenheit and line a baking tray with baking paper
2. In a large bowl, whisk together the coconut oil, egg, vanilla extract, almond milk and stevia
3. Stir the ground almonds, baking powder, chocolate and salt into the wet ingredients until combined
4. Roll the mixture into balls and place them onto your prepared tray
5. Use a fork to gently press down the cookie balls

6. Place the tray into the oven and bake for about 15 minutes or until golden but still a little soft
7. Leave to cool before transferring to an airtight container to store

Nutrition Info: Calories: 19Fat: 17 grams ;Protein: 5 grams ;Total carbs: 7 grams ;Net carbs: 3 grams

Salted Chocolate And Chili Sauce

Servings: 6

Cooking Time:15 Minutes

Ingredients:

- 5 oz 72% cocoa dark chocolate
- 1 ½ cups heavy cream
- ½ tsp sea salt
- ½ tsp chili powder
- 1 tsp Stevia/your preferred keto sweetener

Directions:

1. Place the chocolate and cream into a heatproof bowl and place over a saucepan of boiling water. Stir as the chocolate and cream melt together
2. Add the sea salt, chili and sweetener to the chocolate mixture and stir to combine
3. Transfer the sauce into a pouring jug and keep in the fridge until needed
4. When it's time to use the sauce, heat it up in the microwave to get it back to pouring consistency
5. Serve over keto ice cream, brownies or cake!

Nutrition Info: Calories: 344;Fat: 32 grams;Protein: 3 grams;Total carbs: 9 grams;Net carbs: 5 grams

Avocado Popsicle With Coconut & Lime

Servings: 12

Cooking Time: 1-2 Minutes

Ingredients:

- 4 avocados, peeled, pitted, chopped
- ½ cup erythritol or granular Swerve sweetener
- 3 cups coconut milk
- 4 tablespoons lime juice

Directions:

1. Add avocadoes, erythritol coconut milk and lime juice into a blender.
2. Blend for 30-40 seconds or until smooth. Scrape the sides and blend again.
3. Divide into 12 Popsicle molds. Tap the molds lightly on the countertop. Insert the Popsicle sticks and freeze until firm.
4. To serve: Dip the Popsicle molds in a bowl of warm water for 15 – 20 seconds. The Popsicles will loosen up. Remove from the molds and serve.

Nutrition Info: per Servings: Calories: 91.3 kcal, Fat: 8.g, Carbohydrates: 4.5 g, Protein: 1 g

Dairy-free Pistachio-mint Ice Cream

Servings: 8

Cooking Time:10 Minutes

Ingredients:

- 2 cups full-fat coconut cream
- 3 cups unsweetened almond milk
- 1 ½ cup chopped pistachios
- ⅓ cup finely chopped fresh mint
- 1 tsp Stevia/your preferred keto sweetener
- 4 Tbsp avocado oil

Directions:

1. Use electric beaters to whip the coconut cream until soft, fluffy and thick
2. Carefully fold the almond milk, pistachios, mint, sweetener and avocado oil into the whipped coconut cream (don't worry if the coconut cream deflates, there will still be air hiding in there!)
3. Carefully transfer the mixture into an ice cream container or plastic container, place the lid on and pop it into the freezer
4. Give the ice cream a good stir every hour for the first five hours of freezing time
5. Scoop, serve, enjoy!

Nutrition Info: Calories: 3;Fat: 36 grams ;Protein: 7 grams ;Total carbs: 9 grams;Net carbs: 6 grams

Cinnamon Cake

Servings: 8

Cooking Time: 35minutes

Ingredients:

- For the Cinnamon Filling:
- 3 Tablespoons of Swerve Sweetener
- 2 Teaspoons of ground cinnamon
- For the Cake:
- 3 Cups of almond flour
- ¾ Cup of Swerve Sweetener
- ¼ Cup of unflavoured whey protein powder
- 2 Teaspoon of baking powder
- ½ Teaspoon of salt
- 3 large pastured eggs
- ½ Cup of melted coconut oil
- ½ Teaspoon of vanilla extract
- ½ Cup of almond milk
- 1 Tablespoon of melted coconut oil
- For the cream cheese Frosting:
- 3 Tablespoons of softened cream cheese
- 2 Tablespoons of powdered Swerve Sweetener
- 1 Tablespoon of coconut heavy whipping cream
- ½ Teaspoon of vanilla extract

Directions:

1. Preheat your oven to a temperature of about 325 F and grease a baking tray of 8x8 inch.
2. For the filling, mix the Swerve and the cinnamon in a mixing bowl and mix very well; then set it aside.
3. For the preparation of the cake; whisk all together the almond flour, the sweetener, the protein powder, the baking powder, and the salt in a mixing bowl.
4. Add in the eggs, the melted coconut oil and the vanilla extract and mix very well.
5. Add in the almond milk and keep stirring until your ingredients are very well combined.
6. Spread about half of the batter in the prepared pan; then sprinkle with about two thirds of the filling mixture.
7. Spread the remaining mixture of the batter over the filling and smooth it with a spatula.
8. Bake for about 35 minutes in the oven.
9. Brush with the melted coconut oil and sprinkle with the remaining cinnamon filling.
10. Prepare the frosting by beating the cream cheese, the powdered erythritol, the cream and the vanilla extract in a mixing bowl until it becomes smooth.
11. Drizzle frost over the cooled cake.
12. Slice the cake; then serve and enjoy your cake!

Nutrition Info: Calories: 222;Fat: 19.2g;Carbohydrates: 5.4g;Fiber: 1.5g;Protein: 7.3g

Ginger Cake

Servings: 9

Cooking Time: 20 Minutes

Ingredients:

- ½ Tablespoon of unsalted almond butter to grease the pan
- 4 Large eggs
- ¼ Cup coconut milk
- 2 Tablespoons of unsalted almond butter
- 1 and ½ teaspoons of stevia
- 1 Tablespoon of ground cinnamon
- 1 Tablespoon of natural unweeded cocoa powder
- 1 Tablespoon of fresh ground ginger
- ½ Teaspoon of kosher salt
- 1 and ½ cups of blanched almond flour
- ½ Teaspoon of baking soda

Directions:

1. Preheat your oven to a temperature of 325 F.
2. Grease a glass baking tray of about 8X8 inches generously with almond butter.
3. In a large bowl, whisk all together the coconut milk, the eggs, the melted almond butter, the stevia, the cinnamon, the cocoa powder, the ginger and the kosher salt.

4. Whisk in the almond flour, then the baking soda and mix very well.

5. Pour the batter into the prepared pan and bake for about 20 to 2minutes.

6. Let the cake cool for about 5 minutes; then slice; serve and enjoy your delicious cake.

Nutrition Info: Calories: 1;Fat: 15g;Carbohydrates: 5g;Fiber: 1.9g;Protein: 5g

Berry Chia Pudding

Servings: 4

Cooking Time:10 Minutes

Ingredients:

- 8 Tbsp black chia seeds
- 4 tsp vanilla extract
- 2 tsp Stevia/your preferred keto sweetener
- 1 ½ cups heavy cream
- 1 cup unsweetened almond milk
- 1 cup mixed berries (I use strawberries, raspberries and blueberries)

Directions:

1. Combine all ingredients in a large bowl and leave for about 5 minutes to allow the mixture to start the thickening process as the chia seeds hydrate
2. Divide the mixture into four dessert dishes (or small bowls), cover and place into the fridge overnight
3. Give the pudding a stir before serving with a couple of extra fresh berries on top!

Nutrition Info: Calories: 9;Fat: 40 grams ;Protein: 8 grams ;Total carbs: 11 grams ;Net carbs: 5 grams

Lemon Tart

Servings: 8

Cooking Time:40 Minutes

Ingredients:

- 1 ½ cups ground almonds
- 3 ½ oz butter, melted
- Zest of 1 lemon
- 5 eggs
- 1 cup heavy cream
- ½ cup fresh lemon juice
- 1 ½ tsp Stevia/your preferred keto sweetener

Directions:

1. Preheat the oven to 360 degrees Fahrenheit and thoroughly grease a pie dish with butter
2. Combine the ground almonds, butter and lemon zest. Press the almond mixture into your prepared pie dish. Pop the dish into the oven to bake for 10 minutes
3. Place the eggs, cream, lemon juice and sweetener into a food processor and blitz until combined and smooth
4. Pour the creamy mixture into your prebaked pie crust
5. Place the pie (very carefully!) into the oven and bake for about 20 minutes or until the filling is set but still very slightly wobbly in the center

6. Leave to cool before serving with a dollop of whipped cream!

Nutrition Info: Calories: 345;Fat: 33 grams ;Protein: 9 grams ;Total carbs: 8 grams;Net carbs: 5 grams

Flourless Chocolate Cake

Servings: 6

Cooking Time: 45 Minutes

Ingredients:

- ½ Cup of stevia
- 12 Ounces of unsweetened baking chocolate
- 2/3 Cup of ghee
- 1/3 Cup of warm water
- ¼ Teaspoon of salt
- 4 Large pastured eggs
- 2 Cups of boiling water

Directions:

1. Line the bottom of a 9-inch pan of a spring form with a parchment paper.
2. Heat the water in a small pot; then add the salt and the stevia over the water until wait until the mixture becomes completely dissolved.
3. Melt the baking chocolate into a double boiler or simply microwave it for about seconds.
4. Mix the melted chocolate and the butter in a large bowl with an electric mixer.
5. Beat in your hot mixture; then crack in the egg and whisk after adding each of the eggs.

6. Pour the obtained mixture into your prepared spring form tray.
7. Wrap the spring form tray with a foil paper.
8. Place the spring form tray in a large cake tray and add boiling water right to the outside; make sure the depth doesn't exceed 1 inch.
9. Bake the cake into the water bath for about 45 minutes at a temperature of about 350 F.
10. Remove the tray from the boiling water and transfer to a wire to cool.
11. Let the cake chill for an overnight in the refrigerator.
12. Serve and enjoy your delicious cake!

Nutrition Info: Calories: 295;Fat: 26g;Carbohydrates: 6g;Fiber: 4g;Protein: 8g

Chocolate Chili Pie

Servings: 10

Cooking Time:40 Minutes

Ingredients:

- 1 cup ground almonds
- 3 ½ oz butter, melted
- 2 Tbsp cocoa powder
- Pinch of salt
- 2 tsp Stevia/your preferred keto sweetener
- 2 Tbsp cornstarch

- 2 ½ cups heavy cream
- 7 oz 72% cocoa dark chocolate
- 4 egg yolks in a small bowl
- 2 tsp vanilla extract
- 1 tsp chili powder
- 1 cup heavy cream
- 1 Tbsp cocoa powder
- ½ tsp Stevia/your preferred keto sweetener

Directions:

1. Preheat the oven to 360 degrees Fahrenheit and grease a pie dish with butter
2. Combine the ground almonds, melted butter, cocoa powder and salt
3. Press the almond mixture into your prepared dish (up the sides is best, but don't worry if it's a bit messy and crumbly). Place the dish into your preheated oven to bake for 10 minutes
4. Combine the cornstarch and sweetener with 2 Tbsp of the cream measure to create a slurry (just take the cream out of the 2 ½ cups) and set aside
5. Place the chocolate and remaining cream into a heatproof bowl and place over a saucepan of boiling water and stir as it melts together until smooth

6. Place a small splash of the chocolate/cream mixture into the bowl of egg yolks and whisk to combine thoroughly

7. Transfer the egg yolk mixture into the bowl of chocolate/cream mixture (it should still be over the saucepan of boiling water) and whisk thoroughly

8. Add the vanilla, chili and cornstarch mixture into the bowl and keep whisking as it thickens to a custard-like consistency

9. Pour the custard into your prebaked pie crust and smooth out the top

10. Place the pie into the fridge to set and cool for at least five hours or overnight

11. Make the cream topping just before Servings: beat the cream, cocoa and sweetener until soft and thick. Spread over the pie just before serving!

Nutrition Info: Calories: 247;Fat: 21 grams ;Protein: 4 grams;Total carbs: 9 grams ;Net carbs: 5 grams

www.ingramcontent.com/pod-product-compliance
Lightning Source LLC
Chambersburg PA
CBHW050755030426
42336CB00012B/1823